Weight Loss

Secrets On How To Lose Weight And Feel Great

Table of contents

Introduction

I would like to thank and congratulate you on downloading **"Weight Loss: 10 Pounds In A Week."** You have taken a positive step in finally getting rid of those extra pounds that you have wanted to get rid of. Just think in seven days you are going to be ten pounds lighter. This diet is designed as a short-term diet so once you have reached your weight goal after seven days you need to put yourself back onto a well balanced diet. Just keep in mind that if you follow this diet plan as instructed you will lose the extra pounds that you want to in just seven days! Make sure to prepare yourself and get the foods in that you will need for your diet before you begin. Try and get rid of any foods that may be a temptation for you that you are supposed to avoid during this time.

Making a commitment to yourself that you are going to do this diet is going to be hard to fulfil at times. You must keep the image of you at the end of the seven days as being 10 pounds lighter. Keeping this image in your mind through the diet program is going to help you to get threw those tough moments. Remember nothing worth having ever comes easy, so in order to lose that ten pounds you must stick to the diet in order to obtain the end result of losing ten pounds. Get yourself prepared both mentally and physically for this challenge, make sure that you set a date for when you will begin and finish the diet. This will help to prepare you for this challenge. Tell those around you of your plans and ask them not to come bearing a boxful of doughnuts to share with you on this particular week. If people around you know of your plans they will try and help you to reach your goal by being supportive of you and help encourage you to reach your goal.

Chapter 1
Be Prepared to Lose Weight Fast

We all know that the best way to lose weight is going with a long-term diet and exercise program. But there are those times when we just need to lose some weight as quickly as possible. It could be your wedding is coming up and you want to look at your best for your special day. You may just want to fit into your summer clothes again. Whatever your reason is the information in this book will help you to reach your weight loss goal. We are going to combine innovative diet, exercise and detox plans that are integrated into one program that will get you the end results that you are looking for in a short amount of time. This is a seven-day plan only, it is designed to achieve a specific objective quickly and efficiently it is not meant to be a long-term program. But get ready to have a whole new body transformation in the next seven days.

Talk to Doctor. You should always discuss going on any diet plan with your doctor to make sure that it is going to be safe, you may have health concerns that going on a rapid weight loss program might not be suitable. Your doctor will be able to tell you what kind of weight loss programs are the right ones for you. For example if you have diabetes you can find out from your doctor what foods and how much of them you need to eat to stay healthy. You can also find out what your baseline weight is so that you will have an accurate starting point.

Shopping List. You need to put together a shopping or grocery list of what you are going to be living on for the next seven days. There will be no chips, sweets, candy on this list. You will not have much meat, except chicken breast, so you will not only be losing weight, but saving some money on your grocery shopping.

It is going to be a basically liquid diet that you will be living on. This liquid diet does not include beer or alcoholic beverages. You are going to be eating a lot of soup. Here are the basics of what you will need on your grocery list:

- canned or fresh mushrooms
- canned tomatoes
- carrots
- green onions

- cabbage
- dark green leafy vegetables, spinach, kale
- variety of fresh fruit, including green bananas
- ground cayenne pepper or cayenne capsules
- organic maple syrup
- chicken breast
- green peppers
- celery

For the next few days you are not allowed to eat potatoes and dried beans so make sure to leave them off your list. You can include brown rice, skimmed milk, an unsweetened juice drinks.

Make Soup

How to make soup:

1. Use the first seven items in your grocery list above.
2. Cut them up into small pieces add to soup pot greased with olive oil.
3. Saute lightly and cover with chicken broth (recipe below).
4. Add spices to suit your taste.
5. Cook the soup for about half an hour or until veggies are tender.
6. Make more as needed.

How to make chicken broth:

Take 3 whole chicken breasts, remove, skin, cover with 12 cups of water. Add salt and pepper to taste. Boil for one hour until the breast meat separates from the bones. Remove the chicken meat and refrigerate. Use broth to make soup.

Make your seven day meal plan. During these seven days you will be eating the whole day for these seven days. You must stick to the certain foods that are allowed on certain days of the diet. You can eat as much as you like in that days menu plan, up to six meals a day. This sounds pretty simple does it not?

Here is how the plan will go:

Day 1: Soup and Fruit (any but bananas)

Day 2: Soup and Vegetables, alternate with detox drink (more on this later)

Day 3: Soup, Fruit and vegetables, alternate with detox drink

Day 4: Soup, alternate with detox drink

Day 5: Up to eight bananas, skim milk, plus soup

Day 6: Skinless broiled chicken, soup, vegetables

Day 7: Soup, vegetables, brown rice or whole bread

Keep a Sleep Log. Most of those that are health specialists maintain that getting proper sleep is just as important as making sure to drink enough water daily. Take note of how long you sleep at any given time. Make sure that you are getting enough sleep so that you are not waking up to having a heavy feeling. Most people will need at least eight hours of sleep a day. By keeping a sleep log it will help you to find out what your optimal sleep diet should be.

Chapter 2
Days 1-2 of Diet Program

Day 1 Meals

The first day of your diet is always the easiest because your are still eager and hopeful. You are now all set to begin as you have all the foods that you need to start your diet. You are ready to make the soup that you will need. Stay away from beans, and potatoes during this time, add spices that you like to suit your taste. You may have up to six meals a day if you like, there is no limit on the amount you are allowed to eat, make sure to drink at least eight glasses of water a day or more.

No bananas!

You may find that your meal progression is something like this:

Meal 1: Soup

Meal 2: Apples

Meal 3: Soup and grapes

Meal 4: Oranges

Meal 5: Soup

Meal 6: Grapefruit

If you would prefer to eat more in fewer meals that is up to you, eat in a way that works for you. You may also take vitamins and supplements as long as there is no sugar in them. No protein shakes or protein bars at this time. Black coffee and unsweetened herbal teas are also good liquids for you. Don't take cream or sugar.

If you are doing this diet on your own try and stay away from temptations when others are eating foods that you need to stay away from. Try and eat your meals separately from others to help you to avoid temptation. You may need to be a bit anti-social the next few days in order to keep your resolution strong.

Day 2

Detox and Cleanse to lose Pounds and Gain Energy Overnight

The purpose of this system is to cleanse your system and remove all the unwanted toxins in your body that are clogging up your system, causing you to retain weight. In order to help us to do this we are taking out the hard whole foods that are hard to digest, making the process much easier on your digestive system. In Day 1 of the diet you started the process by eliminating fatty food and meat from your diet. You are now ready to purify your body and your digestive system.

Day 1 of Getting Detoxed. Th process of Detoxification is exactly what it sounds like it is getting rid of the toxins in your body. Your body has a natural elimination system that should be able to do this, but because many of us eat too many processed foods it makes it really hard for our bodies to cope.

The benefits of detoxification and when you are ready to have one:

- When you are feeling fatigued for no particular reason
- looking and feeling haggard even with sufficient sleep
- suffering from skin allergies
- irregular bowel movements
- have a beer gut, even when you are not drinking beer anymore
- have menstrual difficulties that you never experienced before
- feeling confused

Detoxification can help your body as follows:

- it can offer your internal organs a form of relief from the daily inflow of toxic substances
- it can help jump-start you liver into eliminating toxins
- help increase the efficiency of your kidneys, skin and intestines in eliminating waste

- providing healthy nutrients

- help improve blood circulation making it easier to move nutrients around your body

There are many people that recommend detoxification at least once a year, a detoxification program typically takes five days. In this seven day program we are not totally focused on detoxification as an end in itself, but as a means to an end. In this program we are combing the detox program with a more substantial diet to help achieve the goal of losing 10 pounds in the next few days without feeling that you are being deprived.

Making a Detox drink

The most popular detox drink is a combination of organic syrup, cayenne pepper, ginger powder, freshly squeezed lemons. Cayenne pepper and chili powder are both known to help digestion by stimulating the flow of stomach secretions and saliva. You can take it as a capsule if you do not like the taste of cayenne. You need to take at least six eight ounce glasses of this drink a day in order to reap the benefits.

You will need for one glass:

- one twelve ounce glass
- eight ounces of cold drinking water
- two tablespoons of lemon juice
- two tablespoons of cayenne pepper or powdered ginger

Mix all the ingredients in glass.

Day 2 Meals

During the next three days of this program you can choose to alternate your regular meals with the detox drink or have them together. Avoid coffee and cigarettes to get the best results from the detoxification process. You should try and drink at least 64 ounces of water a day.

Your meal progression may look like this:

Meal 1: Soup

Meal 2: Detox drink

Meal 3: Celery and detox drink

Meal 4: Soup and boiled broccoli with detox drink

Meal 5: Tossed salad with lemon vinaigrette (recipe below)

Meal 6: Soup and detox drink

Diet Lemon Vinaigrette

Place the ingredients below in blender:

- half a teaspoon of Dijon mustard
- three quarter teaspoon of salt
- one large garlic clove
- three tablespoons of lemon juice

On day 2 of the diet program you are allowed to eat all the soup and vegetables that you want. The vegetables can be raw or cooked, keep in mind that cooked is easier to digest. Avoid any fruits on day 2 to let your body get used to the effects of the detox drink. You should avoid doing any vigorous exercise as the detox drink can make you feel a little light headed.

Hydrotherapy

Because we are trying to detoxify, you should help the process by enhancing your circulation through hydrotherapy. You can eliminate wastes much faster by increasing your circulation. You can get hydrotherapy in many forms. For now we will just use the shower as our tool. Here is how to do it:

1. Just before bed have a shower in water as hot as you can handle for five minutes.

2. After switch to cold water for 30 seconds.

3. Do this three times then briskly towel yourself dry.

4. Enjoy the best sleep you have ever had!

You have now reached the end of day two, you may feel a bit bloated from all the liquids you have been consuming. Just remember the liquids will be a lot easier to eliminate than solid matter. From this day forward you are going to be eliminating a lot of material. It is not a bad thing don't be alarmed if it may seem and look a little foreign. Much of foods that you eat daily end up getting stuck to your intestines for quite a while. This is very true for white bread and meat. When you are doing your detox all that material will loosen up and will come out. The results may surprise you, but don't worry that just means the system is working.

When you are getting rid of the toxins in your body it is like throwing out the garbage. If you didn't throw out the household garbage it would clutter up the house and it would stink.

Chapter 3
Days 3-4 of Diet Program

To get slimmer faster maximize your calorie burn. You are now well on your way to detoxifying and losing those pounds you want to get rid of. It may be very tempting to check and see what you weigh at this time, but I would suggest that you hold off for a bit. Day 3 is the day that you will start to get your heart rate up.

Exercise Day 1

For many people that are trying to lose weight or would like to lose weight one of the things that they fear most is doing exercise. The truth of the matter is if you want to lose then you are going to have to move off the couch. You need a diet and detox to cleanse and brighten your body. But in order for your body to start burning calories, you are going to have to sweat and stretch it out in some type of aerobic activity.

In order for you to exercise you do not have to go out and buy expensive workout equipment or join a gym. You can start getting your blood running with just what you have around the house. If you are like most people and live a pretty sedentary lifestyle, then you are going to have to work up to the 30 minutes a day you will need to to your cardiovascular system running at a level that is actually going to burn fat. But since you are on a tight schedule a bit of cheating is in the lineup.

If you are going to do exercise do this before you eat your meals to avoid getting cramps.

Normally cardio workouts would start out with 15 minutes a day then working your way up to 30 to 60 minutes without getting too winded. But for this program you will be working out three times a day, building up to a 30 minutes a day workout.

1. Start in the morning before you have breakfast.

2. Pick up again before lunch, for 25 minutes

3. Before dinner, 30 minutes

Think of working out as helping your system to kick start. It may be difficult at first, but it will smooth out in the end. It is low impact exercises, so it will be easy on your joints.

To avoid next morning agonies make sure to warm up and cool down during your workout sessions.

Some important things to remember during exercise sessions.

Remember to breathe in a steady rhythm. Doing this will help oxygenate your blood and eliminate lactic acid from your muscles, and joints that lead to fatigue. Keep making sure to drink lots of water to keep yourself hydrated. You will really have to keep this in mind if you are a person that sweats a lot. Water will also help keep your energy levels up. Don't be pushing yourself too hard. If it has been a long time since you have done any exercise you are going to find that you will tire easily. If you start to feel light headed stop and walk around while breathing deeply.

Step Exercise

Doing step exercise is probably one of the easiest ways to do aerobic exercise. You do not have to leave the house to go to a gym to use special equipment all you need is right in your home.

1. Take your baseline pulse- in the morning before breakfast.

2. Begin to warm up. Warm up for about 60 seconds, walk in place. This can be anywhere— the bathroom, bedroom, living-room etc. This will help loosen your leg muscles. Flap your arms up and down to get the circulation going well.

3. After you feel a bit more limber, go to your staircase and step on the first level one foot after the other. Then step down. Do this for about 15 minutes. You can do it to music or dance steps to make it more entertaining.

4. Walk around for one minute after you have done your step exercise. Your pulse should be elevated, but not racing.

Jump Rope

Another fun exercise at home is using a jump rope. Boxers use a jump rope to build up their stamina, and it doesn't have to be high impacted, you could do it on a carpeted area. Do it slowly but steady for the time you have chosen. If you feel breathless stop jumping, keep moving around, and start again when you feel ready.

Laundry Lifts

You can use your full laundry basket as a form of weights. A full basket of laundry is a great homemade weight. Pick the basket up by squatting and lifting and straightening your legs. This will prevent strain on your back. Once you have lifted it to your head, then lift above your head, then back down. Do this for prescribed time. Make sure to breath regularly. When you are done then it is time to do your laundry.

Getting Detoxed- Day 2

Today you will continue to detoxify, with the requisite 6 to 8 glasses of the detox drink described in Day 2. You can mix in ginger powder instead of cayenne pepper. Also drink 4 glasses of regular water, as you will be losing quite a bit of fluids and other things throughout the day. Don't worry that you find yourself going to the bathroom more often than normal that is just the detox process working.

You may drink your detox hot or cold, add lemon and ginger once hot has cooled down a bit to keep from breaking down nutrients.

Day 3 Meals

On day three of your diet program you are allowed to have fruits, vegetables, and soup. Take it easy on the fruits choose citrus such as oranges, or grapefruits. Favor soup on this day, and boiled vegetables such as squash or broccoli. You can also drink some unsweetened green tea to help with digestion.

No Bananas

Your meal progression may be something like this:

Meal 1: Soup and detox drink

Meal 2: Oranges

Meal 3: Vegetables and Soup and detox drink

Meal 4: Grapefruits

Meal 5: Soup and detox drink

Meal 6: Soup

You may also also want to try a new variation of soup. Here is another soup recipe you can try once you run out of first batch of soup.

- One pack of fat-free vegetable dry soup powder
- two cups of water
- two cups of stock
- two large cans of crushed tomatoes
- tomatoes
- one bunch of spring onions
- green beans
- carrots
- two cubes of bullion
- celery with leaves included

Did you notice that there are no quantities for the vegetables use as much as you like. Make sure to cut the veggies into bite size pieces, put in stock pot. Add salt and pepper to taste and bring to a boil. Reduce heat to simmer cook until veggies are tender. Add spices and herbs, this will be enough soup for two days for one person.

Do not include the following:

- wheat, barley, rye
- nuts
- sugar
- any kind of meat
- butter or oil
- any kind of milk

- beans
- potatoes

You might like to try detoxifying foot bath salts for a nice relaxing soak at the end of a hard stressful day. Now on day three you might be feeling much more energized than normal. Or you could be feeling distracted or irritable. It could take some time for your brain to adjust to the changes that are going on with your body. Don't worry just hang in there and things will work out. You may even have lost up to seven pounds at this point. Just remember not to overdue things because your body is still going through a transition period. Do some relaxation techniques to help loosen your muscles and release those built up toxins in your system. Tomorrow is a new day as part of the your goal to beat the scales

You will find that the detox drink in this program is very simple and easy to make. There is other recipes for detox drinks that you can find online if you get bored or tired of the one with this program. Other detox drinks will work just as well, so if you are looking for a change have a look online for more detox drink recipes.

Day 4

Maintaining Weight Loss and Improving Your Health

At this point in your program you will have eliminated a good portion of toxins, and have also lost some weight too. While your body is adjusting to the new environment, so to speak, you will start to observe a plateau in your weight loss. What ever you do don't be disappointed because a weight loss of 5 to 7 pounds is considered a lot when you are only on the fourth day.

Day 3- Getting Detoxed

The main thing you should be focusing on during day 4 of your program is to start to focus on improving how you physically feel and maintain what you have lost. You may be feeling a little on the low side because you have had no caffeine or sugar for the past three days. You can expect to experience withdrawal symptoms such as:

- menstrual cramps

- muscle pain

- fever

- inability to concentrate

- thirstiness

- nausea

- headaches

- drowsiness

- irritability

You may find that the effects of detoxification can be disheartening. Remember that these are symptoms that are indicative of your body healing itself. Just be patient and hold on it will pass in a couple of days.

Now that you have reached day 4 you are on the last leg of your detox regimen. Most detox programs run between five or more days. By this time you will find that you have gotten the kick-start you need to facilitate elimination. You have now primed your kidneys and liver. So after you finish the 6 to 8 glasses of detox drink, you are done!

Day 4 meals

Because you are trying to destress today you will not do any strenuous exercises today. For your meals you will be having soup alternating with detox drinks. Be ready to take it easy this is like having a pit stop in your progress towards reaching your 10 pound weight loss goal.

Your meal progression will be simple:

Meal 1: Soup

Meal 2: Detox drink

Meal 3: Soup

Meal 4: Detox drink

Meal 5: Soup

Meal 6: Detox drink

You may want to make a thicker soup by adding more veggies to it. It will also help you to feel that it is more of a solid than being mostly liquid.

Sauna

Help yourself to really feel relaxed and treat yourself to a sauna. The steam will help to open your pores. The surface dirt and old sweat will just run off making you feel good and clean. Use a body sponge to help to eliminate dead skin. The heat in the sauna will also help to loosen your muscles and stress will just leak out with sweat. Enjoy a nice hour long session in a sauna, then afterwards to regulate your body temperature take a cool shower after.

If you are not one that likes to visit public spas then perhaps consider a portable steamer that is sold for weight loss. It is basically a large vinyl tent and a plastic seat which dispenses steam. If you don't have that you can still improvise.

You will need:

- a small pail 3/4 full of distilled water
- one portable water heater
- one plastic stool
- a shower curtain

You will be best to do this in the bathroom as it can get wet with the condensation.

Place the water heater in a pail of water and plug it in. Place your stool next to the pail and sit down. Put stool near a wall so you can lean back. Drape the shower curtain around your neck, make sure the pail of water is inside the curtain too. As the water in the pail heats up it will produce steam, and the curtain will trap most of the steam inside. It will escape at your face so it too will get steamed. Relax and let the steam flow over your body for about 15 minutes or until the heat is too uncomfortable for you. Unplug the water heater and relax for five minutes before taking a cold shower. Hang up the curtain so it can drip dry.

If you are not very keen on saunas then you should have a nice hot bath instead. Use some nice essential oils with it such as lavender oil. You will be getting aromatherapy and detoxification at the same time!

If you do have a sauna make sure to have more water today to replace the water you will sweat out during a sauna. Drink up to six glasses of water besides the detox drinks. You should try to do some deep breathing if your tummy feels unsettled or walk around a bit. Enjoy this lazy day for as long as you can because the next three days the pace will be increased. It is not easy making changes even when they are healthy ones, it can have quite traumatic effects, but just stick to it as it will be well worth it in the end.

Chapter 4
Days 5 & 6 of Diet Program

Optimizing Performance to Achieve Better Results

I would like to say to you congratulations on passing the halfway mark to losing those excess pounds! Now that your body is in a pristine state it is time to take advantage of that.

Day 5 Meals

At this point of your program you are going to be feeling the effects of the diet that has next to no carbohydrates, sugar, fat or protein. These are things that your body requires on a regular basis in order for it to function properly. You may be feeling lighted headed or listless at this point in the program. This of course should not be surprising as you are depleting your body's energy sources. It is now time to give your body a boost of energy.

For Day 5 your meals will consist of soup, bananas, and milk. Remember earlier in the program that you were told no bananas? That was because bananas contain starch. It makes it more difficult for you to process than vegetables, and the initial idea was to cleanse your system out as quickly as possible. But at this point in your detox program you need to eat energy-rich foods to counteract the depletion caused by your detox program. Most energy foods are also high in calories and fat.

Bananas on the otherhand are low in fat and calories but high in energy and potassium. That makes it the ideal energy source consistent with weight loss program.

Bananas are also a good source of Vitamin B6 and C, great bonus for your immune system.

You should take bananas 30 minutes before a workout so they can provide you with an energy source. You can also take them before a meal to make it easier for you to digest. You can drink skim milk with your bananas instead of water. You can have as many as eight bananas, but you should have at least one serving of soup. The milk you drink needs to be warm.

Your meal progression may look something like this:

Meal 1: Bananas and warm milk

Meal 2: Soup

Meal 3: Bananas and milk

Meal 4: Soup

Meal 5: Bananas and milk

Meal 6: Soup

The meal regimen of today is of some importance because a second dose of aerobic exercise is needed so you will need the energy to do the workout.

You can try mashing your banana up in the milk to make a smoothie for yourself. You cannot add sugar or artificial sweeteners. Add some cinnamon if you like to spice it up a bit.

Day 2 of Exercise

As before you will gradually be increasing your increments, beginning at 30 minutes for the first session and building up to 45 minutes on the third session. The following are some exercise suggestions. The point is to elevate your pulse and to break out into a sweat. So any activity that you can sustain for 30 minutes and does these two things is fine.

Cycling

You can use a stationary bike or a real bike. If it is a nice day out I would suggest taking out your real bike and getting some fresh air. Make sure that you choose a root that is not going to be hard on your knees. Going for gentle slopes and hills is a good choice especially if you do not bike very often. Bring some water along on your bike ride. Doing an outside bike ride is a great way for you to do some family bonding—make it a family bike ride.

Walking

Get your dog to come out on some good long walks with you. This way you can both get some much needed exercise and he can do his business. If you do not like to go out walking think about getting a treadmill or joining a local gym that has one.

Swimming

Swimming is the best kind of aerobic exercise and it is a fun way to get your heart pumping. You will not be putting strain on your joints and back. Do some slow steady laps for at least 30 minutes, take rest periods when you get tired. Everytime you breathe out you will be releasing toxins out of your body.

Exercise Video

You can watch an exercise video that you can do some aerobic workouts with. You can have some fun dancing with an aerobics class while you get your daily exercise.

Make sure to do warm ups before any of your exercises to make sure that you are not all tightened up. Also include a cool down period in your workout.

At the end of day 5, you will have:

- boosted your energy reserves for the next day
- increased your metabolic rate by doing aerobic exercise
- started taking in carbohydrates while maintaining your weight loss regimen

You are now ready for day 6.

Day 6

Keeping the Will to Win and Maintaining Momentum

You are now arriving on the home stretch of your 7 Days Flat system for losing 10 pounds for a special occasion. You are now on day number 6 it hasn't been all that bad has it?

Well maybe you had some difficult moments going through the process, but you should be proud of yourself that you didn't quit and are still in the program.

Day 6 Meals

There is going to be a bit of a change in your meals for today. Your body is at a point that is is ready for a challenge, and needs the protein, so we will have some boiled chicken with no skin. Remember the chicken used to make broth? It is pretty bland on its own so we will dress it up a bit.

The benefits of chicken for you now are:

- no carbohydrates
- has 110 calories
- is a good source of Vitamin B, selenium, niacin—all good for the immune system
- provides half of the protein you need each day

You can serve as much as you want into your soup. You may also just eat in strips seasoned with salt and pepper. You can also have as much raw or cooked vegetables as you want. You may want to try making a chicken stir fry.

Your meal progression may look similar to this:

Meal 1: Soup

Meal 2: Chicken with vegetables

Meal 3: Soup with vegetables

Meal 4: Soup with chicken

Meal 5: Chicken with vegetables

Meal 6: Soup

Remember for your liquids to take 6 to 8 glasses of water. Unsweetened teas, hot or cold, especially green tea would go well with the chicken.

You will not do any strenuous exercises today but you can use relaxation techniques as the ones mentioned earlier in book such as sauna, hydrotherapy, and breathing exercises.

Check your sleep log

Remember that you should have been keeping notes all along of how you have been sleeping and how much sleep you are getting.

Chapter 5
Day 7 the Final Day of Diet Program!

Reaching your goal...and achieving ongoing success!

This is a wonderful day for you, it is the last day of the program! You have made it to Day 7! You should be so happy and proud of yourself right now. Congrads on having the determination to lose 10 pounds. It is time to wrap this program up!

Exercise for day 3

Now for today you are going to have to do your work out regimen for up to one hour today. You started with 15 minutes on exercise Day 1, and now you are up to 45 minutes. As before you will work your way from 45 minutes to one hour in three increments. You can use any of the forms of exercises that I suggested to you earlier the choice of course is yours. Below are some other exercise suggestions that you might enjoy.

Trampoline!

This is a form of exercise I have recently started using myself, I turn on some of my favorite music—even pipeband music and get bouncing to the beat! It is loads of fun and you get a good workout. You don't have to jump high or exert much effort in this form of exercise. The bouncing motion you are making on the trampoline will signal your body to shift and move aerobically to keep you from losing your balance. Move your torso and arms around to help you to loosen your muscles and stretch. Make sure to breath in through your nose and out through your mouth to release the maximum amount of toxin. Keep some water near by because you will be sweating.

High Tech Workout

If your kids have a game console that has games that you can dance about or box as part of the game this can be a fun way for you to have some bonding time with your kids and get yourself a good fun workout at the same time.

House Cleaning Workout

If you are at home cleaning your house you can still get a workout. You can march on the spot if for example you are doing your dishes, march around as you get things tidied up in your house and before you know it the house is clean and you have gotten your workout for the day

When you lift one foot after the other it will get your blood running no matter how fast you do this. Add some arm rises and deep breathing into it and really get your circulation going. Remember that you need to keep the movement going for at least 30 minutes. You can slow down the pace if you find you are getting tired but keep moving. Try rotating your neck a dozen times clockwise then counterclockwise to help you relieve stress.

Day 7 meals

You have reached the final day of your program this is so exciting for you I am sure, but now to finish off your meals will be a little different today. You are still going to have your soup, which should be taken at least once today. You can also have vegetables, but you will also be allowed to have either whole wheat bread of brown rice, with or without your soup. If you toast the bread it will really go nicely with your soup. Adding some brown rice to your soup can also make it very satisfying. Below are some suggestions for you on how you can make these new culinary additions to your diet help satisfy you. Keep taking your 6 to 8 glasses of water throughout the day.

Bread Dip

A really yummy way to eat bread is to dip it into a balsamic vinegar-oil concoction. Fancy Italian restaurants serve this dip with crunchy bread as an appetizer. The dip itself is so easy to make. All you need to do is to put some balsamic vinegar in a small bowl and add some oil. Cut some whole wheat toasted bread into strips and get dipping! This also goes great with soup too!

Sandwiches

Low-fat salad dressing is just the thing you need to make your sandwich tasty. You can use cucumbers and tomatoes as a filling, maybe even a few strips of boiled chicken breast or half a cup of tuna that has been drained, with or without soup.

Your meal progression may look similar to this:

Meal 1: Toasted bread with soup

Meal 2: Congee

Meal 3: Tuna/Chicken, cucumber, tomato sandwich

Meal 4: Congee

Meal 5: Soup with bread sticks dipped in balsamic-oil dip

Meal 6: Congee

Meditation

Today you might want to try to do some meditation to think about what you have managed to achieve so far. Below is a quote from the ancient Chinese philosopher Lao Tzu:

"Empty your mind of all thoughts. Let your heart be at peace. Watch the turmoil of beings, but contemplate their return. Each separate being in the universe returns to the common source."

Meditation exercises that you might enjoy:

Empty Head

Sometimes the build up of stress can make you feel that you cannot breath. In this exercise the purpose is to clear your mind of all thought.

1. Find a nice cool, dark place.

2. Get into a comfortable sitting position on the floor, perhaps on a cushion. Many find that sitting cross-legged is the most comfortable position.

3. Set your hands on top of your knees with palms facing up, keep your hands straight without tensing them.

4. Breathe slowly with your mouth closed, have your tongue touching the back of your upper teeth.

5. Close your eyes and let your thoughts flow.

6. Imagine blowing each thought as it comes away with each breath you exhale.

7. Visualize and empty room and listen to your breath as it comes in and out.

8. Do this for five minutes.

At the end of it you may not achieve an empty head, but you will feel much more relaxed!

Stream of thought

- find a clean and quiet place
- sit in a position that is comfortable for you
- close your eyes and concentrate on the darkness
- let your thoughts flow without interruption
- if there is something that you want to focus on repeat the word in your head
- stay in this position for ten minutes

Time to Do the Weigh In

This is the time when you have a drum roll just before you weigh in. Remember that you established your baseline weight on day one of the program? Well now you will find out exactly how much weight you have lost in this past week.

If you stuck completely to the instructions and guidelines of the program you should have lost 10 pounds. If you have a pound here or there on either side of your goal keep in mind that individual body chemistry can be a major factor in your result. What this basically means is that every person will react in different ways to this program. On the average people lose ten pounds on this program. You should also have lost a couple of inches all over your body. I just want to say congratulations on making it to the end of your goal and sticking through it from beginning to end. You at this moment should be very proud and happy that you were able to accomplish this feat. Accomplishing this goal is not only going to have you looking and feeling great it is also going to build up your self-confidence level. I wish you great success in life and now that you have reached this goal you can begin to plan what your next goal will be!

Planning Your Maintenance Regimen

You need to make a new grocery list as part of planning your maintenance regimen. This is going to help you to come back to a normal balanced diet. In this new diet plan you may now include coffee, potatoes, sugar, and all the other food items that were eliminated from your diet. But in order for you to maintain your ideal weight you must continue to avoid foods that are high in fat, sugar, and bad carbohydrates, as well as other bad habits like missing meals. Below is a list of food to avoid:

- white bread and crackers
- sugar
- alcoholic drinks, sodas, sweetened beverages
- fast food and high fat snack foods
- food high in fat
- fried foods

You should also continue to do some form of aerobic exercise at least three times per week.

All of the detoxifying activities described in this program can be used on a daily basis, save for the detox drink. You can go on detoxification programs every six months or so if you feel that you really need it. If you are maintaining a healthy regimen, once a year should be more than enough to do a detoxification program.

Well that is it you have achieved your short term goal and lost the weight. For the long term I hope that you will begin to live a more healthy lifestyle. Now you can rest and enjoy the accomplishment that you have achieved in the past week, sit back and enjoy the moment. This is one known as a natural high—achieving goals that you set out for yourself will give you this wonderful high feeling of peace and contentment. Congrads on sticking through the program to the end!

Conclusion

I hope that you achieved your personal weight loss goal by using this program. If you followed it and stuck with the instructions and guidelines I have no doubt that you have been successful. Now you can be proud of yourself for achieving this short-term goal. Now it is up to you to keep up a balanced diet and exercise program that is going to benefit you in the long-term with health and happiness. I wish you great success in your personal journey to achieving long-term health and happiness. Just remember when you put your mind to a goal you know that you can accomplish it!

Thanks again for downloading my book if you enjoyed it and found it helpful please leave a small review of it at Amazon it would be most helpful and appreciated by me! Take care and good luck on your next personal goal—you can do it!

www.ingramcontent.com/pod-product-compliance
Lightning Source LLC
Chambersburg PA
CBHW070829260726
48654CB00024B/655